The Quick and Easy Keto Diet Cookbook for Beginners

Boost your Metabolism and your Health with this Collection of Keto Desserts

Sammy Owens

Contents

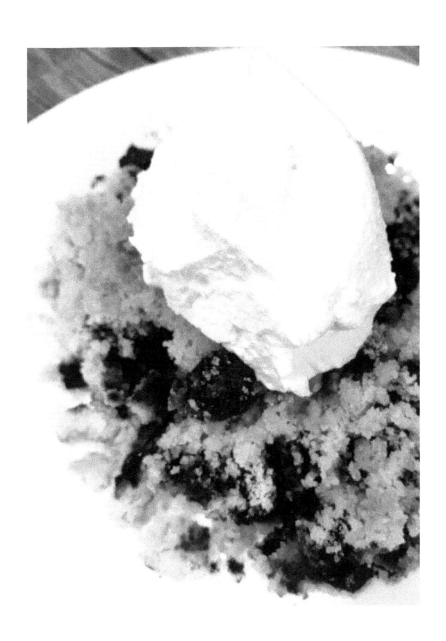

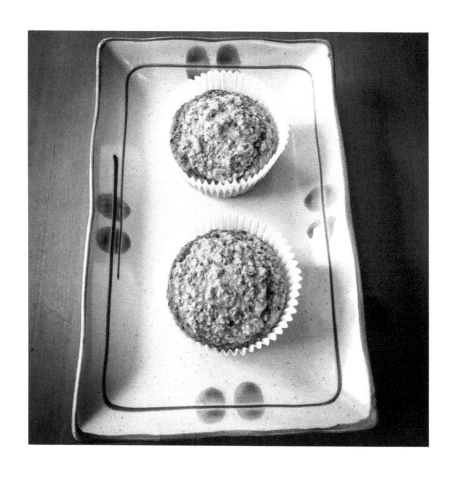

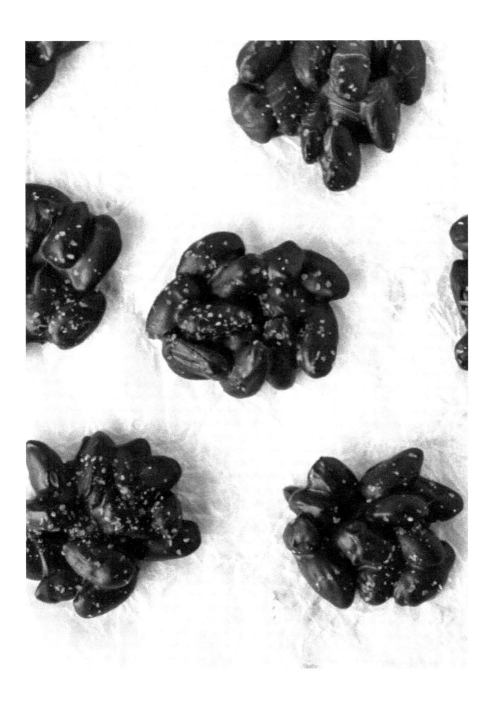

Raspberry And Cashew Balls

Servings: 14

Cooking Time: 0 Minutes

Ingredients:

- 1⅓ Cup of raw cashews or almonds
- ¼ Cup of cashew or almond butter
- 2 Tablespoons of coconut oil
- 2 Pitted Medjool dates, pre-soaked into hot water for about 10 minutes
- ½ Teaspoon of vanilla extract
- ¼ Teaspoon of kosher salt
- ½ Cup of freeze-dried and lightly crashed raspberries
- ⅓ Cup of chopped dark chocolate

Directions:

1. In a high-powered blender or a Vitamix; combine the cashews or almonds with the butter, the coconut oil, the Medjool dates, the vanilla extract and the salt and pulse on a high speed for about to 2 minutes or until the batter starts sticking together.
2. Pulse in the dried raspberries and the dark chocolate until your get a thick mixture.
3. With a tablespoon or a small cookie scoop, divide the mixture into balls of equal size.

4. Arrange the balls in a container or a zip-top bag in a refrigerator for about 2 weeks or just serve and enjoy your delicious cashew balls!

Nutrition Info: Calories: 108.2| Fat: 7.4 g;Carbohydrates: 9g;Fiber: 1.3g;Protein: 3 g

Salted Chocolate And Hazelnut Balls

Servings: 15

Cooking Time:10 Minutes

Ingredients:

- 5 oz butter, melted
- ½ cup ground almonds
- 1 cup finely chopped toasted hazelnuts
- 4 oz full fat ricotta cheese
- 1 tsp sea salt
- ½ tsp Stevia/your preferred keto sweetener
- 3 Tbsp unsweetened cocoa powder

Directions:

1. Line a baking tray with baking paper
2. Combine all ingredients in a large bowl until completely combined
3. Roll the mixture into balls and place into your lined tray
4. Place the tray into the fridge for an hour to allow the balls to set and harden
5. Store the balls in an airtight container in the fridge until needed

Nutrition Info: Calories: 152;Fat: 15 grams ;Protein: 3 grams ;Total carbs: 3 grams ;Net carbs: 1 gram

Coconut Keto Bombs

Servings: 14

Cooking Time: 0 Minutes

Ingredients:

- 1 and ½ cups of walnuts or any type of nuts of your choice
- ½ Cup of shredded coconut
- ¼ Cup of coconut butter + 1 additional tablespoon of extra coconut butter
- 2 Tablespoons of almond butter
- 2 Tablespoons of chia seeds
- 2 Tablespoons of flax meal
- 2 Tablespoons of hemp seeds
- 1 Teaspoon of cinnamon
- ½ Teaspoon of vanilla bean powder
- ¼ Teaspoon of kosher salt
- 2 Tablespoons of cacao nibs
- For the chocolate drizzle
- 1 Oz of unsweetened chocolate, chopped
- ½ Teaspoon of coconut oil

Directions:

1. In the mixing bowl of your food processor, combine the walnuts with the coconut butter; the almond butter, the chia seeds, the flax meal, the hemp seeds,

the cinnamon, the vanilla bean powder, the shredded coconut and the chopped; then drizzle with the coconut oil.

2. Pulse your ingredients for about 1 to minutes or until the mixture starts breaking down.

3. Keep processing your mixture until it starts to stick together; but just be careful not to over mix.

4. Add in the cacao nibs and pulse until your ingredients.

5. With a small cookie scoop or simply with a tablespoon, divide the mixture into pieces of equal size.

6. Use both your hands to toll the mixture into balls; then arrange it over a platter.

7. Store the balls in an airtight container or place it in the freezer for about 15 minutes.

8. Serve and enjoy your delicious balls!

Nutrition Info: Calories: 164| Fat: 14 g;Carbohydrates: 5.;Fiber: 2g;Protein: 4 g

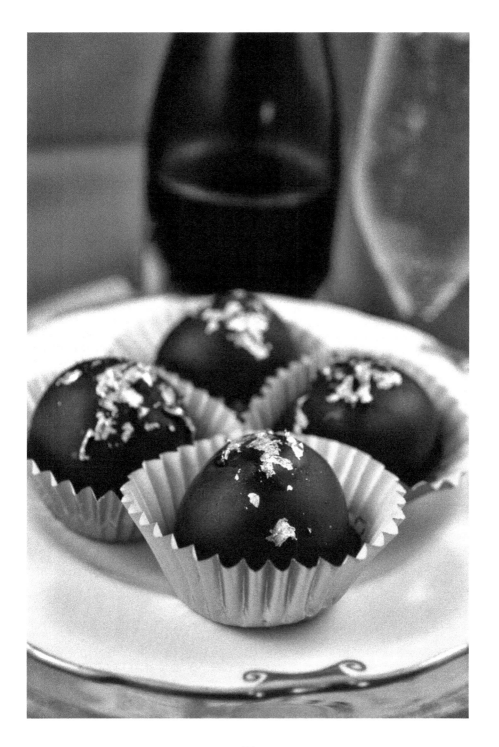

Chocolate Vanilla Truffles

Servings: 20

Cooking Time:15 Minutes

Ingredients:

- 7 oz 72% cocoa dark chocolate
- 1 cup heavy cream
- 1 Tbsp vanilla extract
- ½ tsp Stevia/your preferred keto sweetener
- ½ cup unsweetened cocoa powder (for rolling)

Directions:

1. Place the chocolate and cream into a heatproof bowl and place over a saucepan of boiling water
2. Stir as the chocolate melts into the cream
3. Stir the vanilla and sweetener into the chocolate/cream mixture and leave to cool completely
4. Spread the cocoa powder into the bottom of a shallow bowl
5. Use a metal dessert spoon to scoop small portions of chocolate mixture, very quickly roll the mixture into rough balls (they can be raggedy, truffles aren't meant to be totally round and smooth!)
6. Roll the balls in the cocoa powder until they're completely coated

7. Place the balls onto a plate and pop into the fridge to harden for an hour before serving or packing into an airtight container

Nutrition Info: Calories: 103;Fat: grams ;Protein: 1 gram;Total carbs: 7 grams ;Net carbs: 6 grams

Blueberry Fat Bombs

Servings: 30

Cooking Time: 0 Minutes

Ingredients:

- 4 Oz of soft goat's cheese
- ½ Cup of fresh blueberries
- 1 Cup of almond flour
- 1 Teaspoon of vanilla extract
- ½ Cup of pecans
- ½ Teaspoon of stevia
- ¼ Cup of unsweetened shredded coconut

Directions:

1. Process the goat cheese with the fresh blueberries, the almond flour, the vanilla extract, the pecans, the stevia and the unsweetened shredded coconut in a food processor and process very well
2. Roll the mixture into about 30 small fat bombs
3. Pour the coconut flakes in a bowl and lightly roll each of the fat bombs into the shredded coconut
4. Serve and enjoy your delicious fat bombs!

Nutrition Info: Calories: 49;Fat: g;Carbohydrates: 1g;Fiber: 1g;Protein: 2.3 g

Lemon And Poppy Seed Fat Bombs

Servings: 18

Cooking Time: 1 Hour

Ingredients:

- 8 oz cream cheese, softened
- 3 tbsp erythritol
- 1 tbsp poppy seeds
- 1 lemon, zested
- 4 tbsp sour cream
- 2 tbsp lemon juice

Directions:

1. Add everything to a bowl and beat them together using a hand mixer on low speed for 3 minutes.
2. Divide this mixture into a mini cupcake tray layered with cupcake liners and place it in the refrigerator for 1 hour.
3. Serve.

Nutrition Info: Calories 113 Total Fat 9 g Saturated Fat 0.2 g Cholesterol 1.7 mg Sodium 13mg Total Carbs 6.5 g Sugar 1.8 g Fiber 0.7 g Protein 7.5 g

Quick Bread In The Frying Pan

Servings: 4-6

Cooking Time: 20 Minutes

Ingredients:

- ⅓ cup + 1 tbsp almond flour
- 1 ½ tbsp psyllium
- 3 eggs
- ½ cup yogurt
- ½ cup grated cheese
- 1 tsp baking powder
- 2 tsp flax seeds
- 2 tsp sesame seeds
- 1 tbsp coconut oil (for frying)
- 1 tbsp pumpkin seeds (for decoration)
- A pinch of salt

Directions:

1. In a bowl, beat the eggs by a mixer until uniformity. Add grated cheese, yogurt, and dry ingredients. Mix it all. Leave for minutes.
2. Grease the frying pan, and lay out the dough. Sprinkle with pumpkin seeds.
3. Fry on low heat for 7 minutes on each side. Serve warm.

Nutrition Info: Per Servings: Calories: 91 Fats: 12.3 g Carbs: 3.6 g Proteins: 21 g

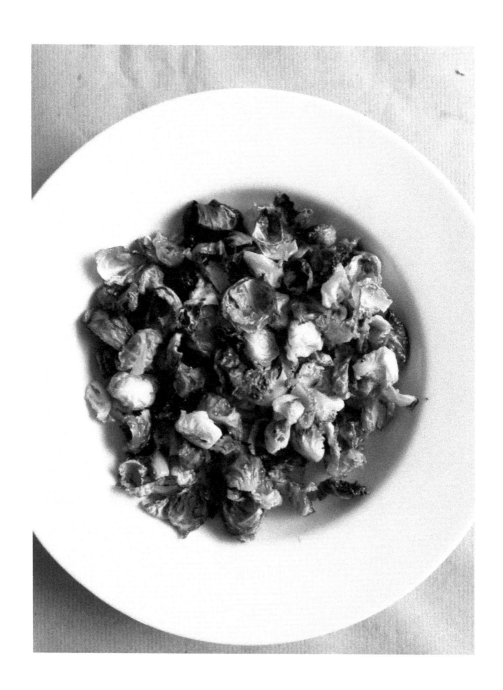

Brussels Sprouts Chips

Servings: 6

Cooking Time: 15 Minutes

Ingredients:

- 1 pound Brussels sprouts, washed and dried
- 2 tbsp extra virgin olive oil
- 1 tsp kosher salt

Directions:

1. Preheat your oven at 400 degrees F.
2. After peeling the sprouts off the stem, discard the outer leaves of the Brussel sprouts.
3. Separate all the leaves from one another and place them on a baking sheet.
4. Toss them with oil and salt thoroughly to coat them well.
5. Spread the leaves out on two greased baking sheets then bake them for 1minutes until crispy.
6. Serve.

Nutrition Info: Calories 188 Total Fat 3 g Saturated Fat 2.2 g Cholesterol 101 mg Sodium 54 mg Total Carbs 3 g Sugar 1.3 g Fiber 0.6 g Protein 5 g

Cheesy Taco Bites

Servings: 12

Cooking Time: 10minutes

Ingredients:

- 2 Cups of Packaged Shredded Cheddar Cheese
- 2 Tablespoon of Chilli Powder
- 2 Tablespoons of Cumin
- 1 Teaspoon of Salt
- 8 Teaspoons of coconut cream for garnishing
- Use Pico de Gallo for garnishing as well

Directions:

1. Preheat your oven to a temperature of about 350 F.
2. Over a baking sheet lined with a parchment paper, place 1 tablespoon piles of cheese and make sure to a space of inches between each.
3. Place the baking sheet in your oven and bake for about 5 minutes.
4. Remove from the oven and let the cheese cool down for about 1 minute; then carefully lift up and press each into the cups of a mini muffin tin.
5. Make sure to press the edges of the cheese to form the shape of muffins mini.
6. Let the cheese cool completely; then remove it.

7. While you continue to bake the cheese and create your cups.

8. Fill the cheese cups with the coconut cream, then top with the Pico de Gallo.

9. Serve and enjoy your delicious snack!

Nutrition Info: Calories: 73;Fat: 5g;Carbohydrates: 3g;Fiber: 1g;Protein: 4g

Rye Crackers

Servings: 10

Cooking Time: 15 Minutes

Ingredients:

- 1 cup rye flour
- 23 cup bran
- 2 tsp baking powder
- 3 tbsp vegetable oil
- 1 tsp liquid malt extract
- 1 tsp apple vinegar
- 1 cup water
- Salt to taste

Directions:

1. Combine flour with bran, baking powder and salt.
2. Pour in oil, vinegar and malt extract. Mix well.
3. Knead the dough, gradually adding the water.
4. Divide and roll it out with a rolling pin about 0.1 inch thick.
5. Cut out (using a knife or cookie cutter) the crackers of square or rectangle shape.
6. Bake at 390°F for 12–15 minutes.

Nutrition Info: Per Servings: Calories 80 Total carbs 10.4 g Protein 1.1 g Total fat 4.3 g

Keto Mug Bread

Servings:1

Cooking Time: 2 Minutes

Ingredients:

- 13 cup Almond Flour
- ½ tsp Baking Powder
- ¼ tsp Salt
- 1 Whole Egg
- 1 tbsp Melted Butter

Directions:

1. Mix all ingredients in a microwave-safe mug.
2. Microwave for 90 seconds.
3. Cool for 2 minutes.

Nutrition Info: Per Servings: Fat: 37 g. Protein: 15 g. Carbs: 8 g.

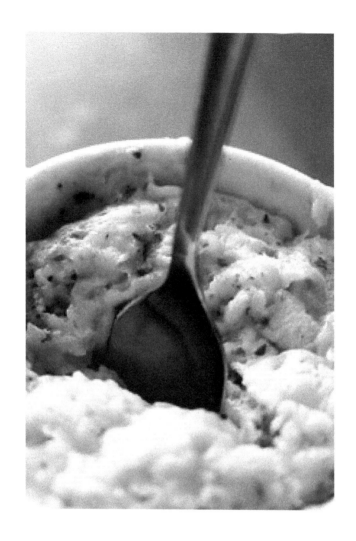

Ketogenic Madeleine

Servings: 12

Cooking Time: 15 Minutes

Ingredients:

- 2 Large pastured eggs
- ¾ Cup of almond flour
- 1 and ½ Tablespoons of Swerve
- ¼ Cup of cooled, melted coconut oil
- 1 Teaspoon of vanilla extract
- 1 Teaspoon of almond extract
- 1 Teaspoon of lemon zest
- ¼ Teaspoon of salt

Directions:

1. Preheat your oven to a temperature of about 350 F.
2. Combine the eggs with the salt and whisk on a high speed for about 5 minutes.
3. Slowly add in the Swerve and keep mixing on high for 2 additional minutes.
4. Stir in the almond flour until it is very well-incorporated; then add in the vanilla and the almond extracts.
5. Add in the melted coconut oil and stir all your ingredients together.

6. Pour the obtained batter into equal parts in a greased Madeleine tray.
7. Bake your Ketogenic Madeleine for about 13 minutes or until the edges start to have a brown color.
8. Flip the Madeleines out of the baking tray.
9. Serve and enjoy your madeleines!

Nutrition Info: Calories: 87;Fat: 8.1g;Carbohydrates: 3g;Fiber: 2g;Protein: 8g

Buns With Zucchini

Servings: 8

Cooking Time: 45 Minutes

Ingredients:

- ½ cup almond flour
- 5 eggs
- 2 tbsp sucralose
- ½ cup grated cheese
- 1 zucchini
- 3 tbsp flax seeds
- ½ cup sunflower seeds
- 2 tbsp psyllium
- 1 tsp baking powder
- ½ tsp salt
- 1 tbsp dried oregano

Directions:

1. The oven to be preheated to 200°C (400°F).
2. Grate the zucchini on a fine grater and squeeze out mass, removing excess liquid. Season with salt.
3. In a bowl, beat the eggs by a mixer for 2 minutes until dense foam. Add grated cheese, zucchini, and dry ingredients. Mix well. Leave the dough for 8 minutes.
4. Divide the dough into round buns. Bake in the oven for 25 minutes.

Nutrition Info: Per Servings: Calories: 11 Fats: 10 g Carbs: 2.9 g Proteins: 12.2 g

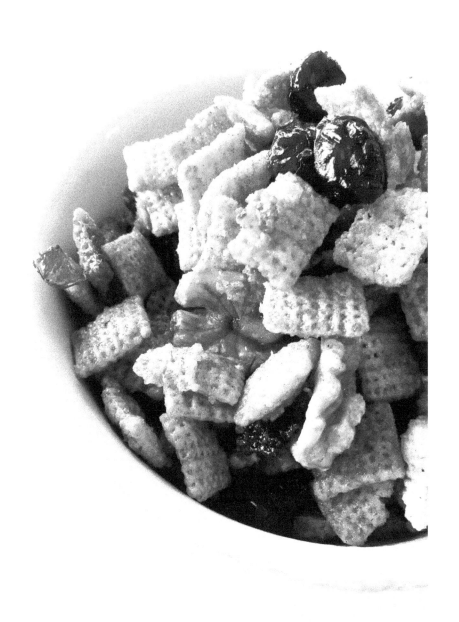

Nut Squares

Servings: 10

Cooking Time: 10 Minutes

Ingredients:

- 2 Cups of almonds, pumpkin seeds, sunflower seeds and walnuts
- ½ Cup of desiccated coconut
- 1 Tablespoon of chia seeds
- ¼ Teaspoon of salt
- 2 Tablespoons of coconut oil
- 1 Teaspoon of vanilla extract
- 3 Tablespoons of almond or peanut butter
- 1/3 Cup of Sukrin Gold Fiber Syrup

Directions:

1. Line a square baking tin with a baking paper; then lightly grease it with cooking spray
2. Chop all the nuts roughly; then slightly grease it too, you can also leave them as whole
3. Mix the nuts in a large bowl; then combine them in a large bowl with the coconut, the chia seeds and the salt
4. In a microwave-proof bowl; add the coconut oil; then add the vanilla, the coconut butter or oil, the almond butter and the fiber syrup and microwave the mixture for about 30 seconds

5. Stir your ingredients together very well; then pour the melted mixture right on top of the nuts

6. Press the mixture into your prepared baking tin with the help of the back of a measuring cup and push very well

7. Freeze your treat for about 1 hour before cutting it

8. Cut your frozen nut batter into small cubes or squares of the same size

9. Serve and enjoy!

Nutrition Info: Calories: 268;Fat: 22g;Carbohydrates: 14g;Fiber: 1g;Protein: 7g

Focaccia

Servings: 2-4

Cooking Time: 35 Minutes

Ingredients:

- 1 package bread baking mass
- 1 ⅓ cup water
- 2 tbsp olive oil
- ¼ cup olives
- ½ tsp sea salt
- 1 tsp dry rosemary

Directions:

1. Mix the dough from the bread mass, water, and olive oil.
2. Cover the baking sheet with parchment.
3. Roll out the dough on a baking into a flat cake. Decorate with olives, sprinkle with salt and rosemary.
4. Bake in the oven at 200°C (0°F) for 20 minutes.
5. Important! You can use dried tomatoes, cheese, bacon, garlic, and mushrooms as a decorating.

Nutrition Info: Per Servings: Calories: 78 Fats: 10 g Carbs: 5 g Proteins: 8 g

Carrot Buns

Servings: 8

Cooking Time: 35 Minutes

Ingredients:

- ½ cup almond flour
- ½ cup chopped cheese
- 5 eggs
- ½ cup sunflower seeds
- 2 carrots
- 3 tbsp chia seeds
- 2 tbsp psyllium
- 1 tsp baking powder
- ½ tsp salt

Directions:

1. The oven to be preheated to 200°C (400°F).
2. Grate the carrots on a fine grater. In a bowl, beat the eggs by a mixer for minutes until dense mass. Add grated cheese, carrot puree, and dry ingredients. Mix until uniformity. Leave the dough for 8 minutes.
3. Make the round buns and lay out them on the baking sheet covered with parchment. Ensure that it is baked for 20 minutes.

Nutrition Info: Per Servings: Calories: 85 Fats: 12 g Carbs: 3.2 g Proteins: 9 g

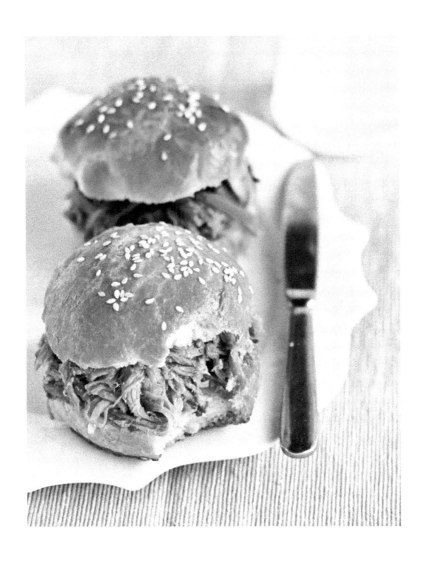

Almond Buns

Servings: 4

Cooking Time: 15 Minutes

Ingredients:

- ¼ cup almond flour
- 1 egg
- 2 tbsp butter
- 1 ½ tsp baking powder

Directions:

1. The oven to be preheated to 200°C (400°F).
2. In a bowl, mix the flour, the melted butter, and the egg. Add baking powder to the mass and mix well to get an airy dough.
3. Lay out the dough into silicone forms for cupcakes and bake in the oven for 10 minutesutes. Leave buns in the oven for minutesutes.

Nutrition Info: Per Servings: Calories: 55 Fats: 8 g Carbs: 0.9 g Proteins: 5 g

Bread With Feta And Basil

Servings: 10-12

Cooking Time: 65 Minutes

Ingredients:

- ⅔ cup almond flour
- ¼ cup coconut flour
- 3.5 oz feta
- 2 tbsp coconut oil
- 7 eggs
- 2 tbsp psyllium
- 1 tbsp stevia
- 2 tsp baking powder
- 2 tsp dry basil

Directions:

1. The oven to be preheated to 0°C (375°F).
2. In a bowl, beat the eggs by a mixer until uniformity. Chop feta, and add melted coconut oil. Add the cheese to the egg mass, and mix it all.
3. In another bowl, mix all the dry ingredients, and add to the cheese base. Leave the dough for 10 minutes.
4. Cover the baking sheet with parchment. Make the bread and lay out on the baking sheet. Bake in the oven for 55 minutes.

Nutrition Info: Per Servings: Calories: 70 Fats: 6 g Carbs: 1.6 g Proteins: 7.3 g

Keto Sugar Free Candies

Servings: 12

Cooking Time: 0 Minutes

Ingredients:

- 4 Oz of Coconut Oil, melted
- 4.5 Oz of Shredded, unsweetened Coconut
- 1 Teaspoon of Stevia
- 3 Oz of Erythritol powder
- 1 Large egg white
- 1 Teaspoon of vanilla extract
- 3 Drops of Red Food Colouring
- ½ Teaspoon of Strawberry Extract

Directions:

1. In a large bowl, mix all together the erythritol, the shredded coconut, the stevia and the vanilla with a hand blender on a low heat.
2. Melt the coconut oil in a small saucepan over a low heat.
3. Add the oil to the shredded coconut mixture and combine very well.
4. Add in the egg white and mix; then combine half of the mixture into a square dish of about 8 squares and set it aside.

5. Add the strawberry essence and the food colouring and strawberry essence to the remaining mixture and mix very well.

6. Press the mixture right top of the white mixture into the square dish and set it aside in the fridge for about 1 hour.

7. When your coconut ice is perfectly set, cut it into 16 pieces.

8. Serve and enjoy!

Nutrition Info: Calories: 11Fat: 12g;Carbohydrates: 2g;Fiber: 1g;Protein: 3g

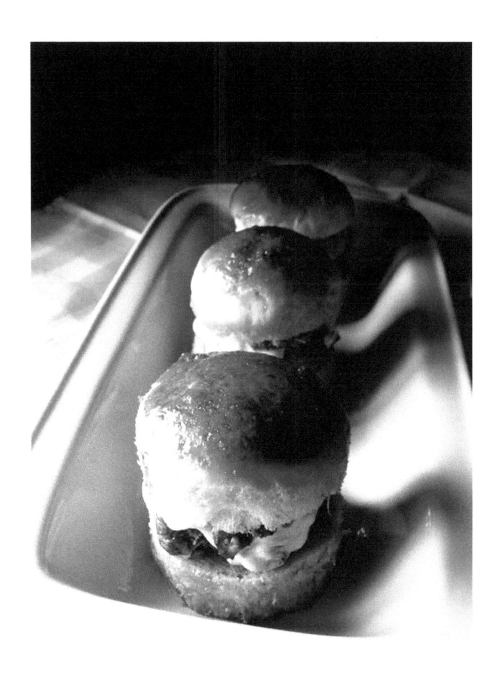

Buns With Walnuts

Servings: 4

Cooking Time: 40 Minutes

Ingredients:

- 5 eggs
- 3 tbsp almond flour
- 3 tbsp coconut flour
- 1 ½ tbsp psyllium
- 2 tbsp butter
- ½ cup yogurt
- ½ cup grated parmesan
- 2 tsp baking powder
- ½ cup walnuts
- ½ tbsp cuminutes (for decoration)

Directions:

1. The oven to be preheated to 0°C (375°F).
2. In a bowl, beat the eggs by a mixer until uniformity. Add soft butter, dry ingredients, yogurt, and crushed walnuts. Mix well. Add the grated parmesan. Leave the dough for 10 minutes.
3. Make the round buns with wet hands, and lay out them on the baking sheet covered with parchment.
4. Season with cuminutes and bake in the oven for 20 minutes.

Nutrition Info: Per Servings: Calories: 16 Fats: 23.1 g Carbs: 4.5 g Proteins: 18 g

Coconut Snack Bars

Servings: 13

Cooking Time: 0 Minutes

Ingredients:

- 2 Cups of coconut flakes
- ¾ Cup of melted coconut oil
- 1 and ½ cups of macadamia nuts
- 1 large scoop of vanilla protein powder
- ¼ Cup of unsweetened dark chocolate chips

Directions:

1. Gather the coconut flakes with the melted coconut oil, the macadamia nuts, the vanilla protein powder and the dark chocolate chips in a large bowl and mix very well.
2. Line an 8×8 baking tray with a parchment paper.
3. Process the macadamia nuts with the coconut oil in a food processor until it becomes smooth.
4. Pour the batter into a pan and freeze it for about 30 minutes.
5. Cut the frozen batter into bars with a sharp knife into your preferred size.
6. Serve and enjoy your Ketogenic treat or store it and serve it whenever you want.

Nutrition Info: Calories: 213.Fat: 20g;Carbohydrates: 6g;Fiber: 2 g;Protein: 4g

Keto Donuts

Servings: 4

Cooking Time: 0 Minutes

Ingredients:

- For the donut ingredients:
- ½ Cup of sifted almond flour
- 3 to 4 tablespoons of coconut milk
- 2 Large eggs
- 2 to 3 tablespoons granulated of stevia
- 1 Teaspoon of Keto-friendly baking powder
- 1 Heap teaspoon of apple cider vinegar
- 1 Pinch of salt
- 1 and ½ Tablespoon of sifted cacao powder
- 3 Teaspoons of Ceylon cinnamon
- 1 Teaspoon of powdered vanilla bean
- 1 Tablespoon of grass-fed ghee
- 2 Tablespoons of Coconut oil for greasing
- For the Icing Ingredients:
- 4 Tablespoons of melted coconut butter with 1 to 2 teaspoons of coconut oil
- Optional garnishing ingredients: edible rose petals, or shredded cacao

Directions:

1. Preheat the oven to a temperature of about 350 degrees.
2. Grease a donut tray with the coconut oil.
3. Stir all together the sifted almond flour with the coconut milk, eggs, the granulated of stevia, the Keto-friendly baking powder, the apple cider vinegar, the salt, the sifted cocoa powder, the Ceylon cinnamon, the powdered vanilla bean and the grass-fed ghee.
4. Mix your donut ingredients until they are evenly combined.
5. Divide the obtained batter into the donut moulds making sure to fill each to ¾ full.
6. Bake for about 8 minutes; then remove the tray from the oven and carefully transfer it to a wire rack.
7. Serve and enjoy your donut or top it with the icing and the garnish of your choice.
8. Serve and enjoy your delicious treat!

Nutrition Info: Calories: 122;Fat: 6.8g;Carbohydrates: 13.5g;Fiber: 2.3g;Protein: 3g

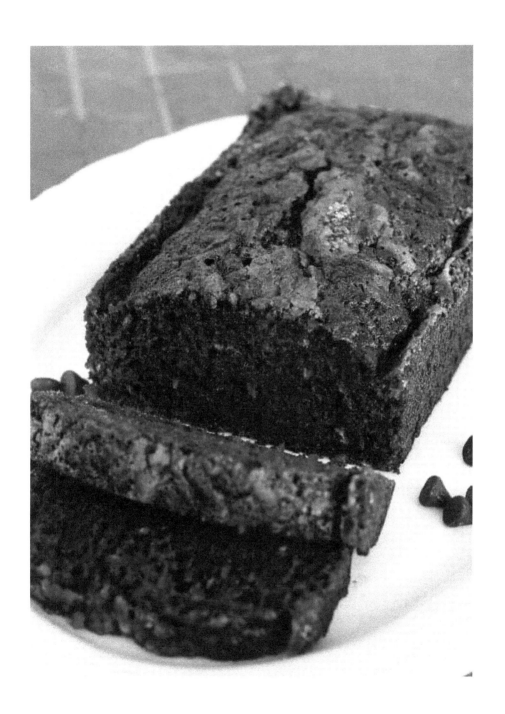

Chocolate And Zucchini Bread

Servings: 10-12

Cooking Time: 50 Minutes

Ingredients:

- ¾ cup + 1 tbsp almond flour
- 1 zucchini
- 1 tsp baking powder
- 2 tbsp cocoa powder
- ½ tsp cinnamon
- 2 eggs
- ¼ cup yogurt
- 3.5 oz soft coconut oil
- ½ tsp vanilla
- 1 tsp balsamic vinegar
- 1 tbsp chopped almonds
- 3 tbsp liquid stevia
- A pinch of salt

Directions:

1. The oven to be preheated to 0°C (356°F).
2. Chop zucchini until uniformity, and add almonds. In a bowl, combine the flour, baking powder, cinnamon, cocoa powder, and salt.

3. In another bowl, beat the eggs; add coconut oil, yogurt, vanilla, stevia, and vinegar. Mix it all. Add zucchini and dry ingredients to the egg mass. Mix well.

4. Grease the baking sheet. Lay out the dough and bake in the oven for 35 minutes. Cool the bread and put it on the plate.

Nutrition Info: Per Servings: Calories: 89 Fats: 9.7 g Carbs: 2.7 g Proteins: 3 g

Buns With Poppy Seeds

Servings: 1-2

Cooking Time: 10 Minutes

Ingredients:

- 1 tbsp almond flour
- 1 tbsp coconut flour
- 1 tsp butter
- ½ tsp baking powder
- 1 egg
- 1 tbsp cream
- ½ tsp poppy seeds
- A pinch of salt

Directions:

1. Grease the silicone baking form.
2. Add the egg and cream. Mix everything until uniformity.
3. Pour the dough into a form and put in a microwave for minutes.
4. Cut ready buns in half and fry in a dry frying pan for 1 minutesute.

Nutrition Info: Per Servings: Calories: 89 Fats: 13 g Carbs: 3 g Proteins: 7.1 g

Nuts Bread

Servings: 10-12

Cooking Time: 75 Minutes

Ingredients:

- 1 cup almond flour
- 3 eggs
- ¼ cup olive oil
- 2 oz Brazil nuts
- 2 oz hazelnuts
- 2 oz walnuts
- ½ cup sesame seeds
- 2 tbsp flax seeds
- 2 tbsp pumpkin seeds
- A pinch of salt

Directions:

1. The oven to be preheated to 0°C (338°F).
2. Crush all the nuts in a blender until uniformity.
3. In a bowl, mix the dry ingredients. Add whipped eggs and butter. Mix it all.
4. Grease the baking dish. Lay out the dough. Bake in the oven for 60 minutes.

Nutrition Info: Per Servings: Calories: 103 Fats: 13.1 g Carbs: 1.6 g Proteins: 6.g

Hazelnut Breadstick With Seeds

Servings: 10

Cooking Time: 40 Minutes

Ingredients:

- ½ cup hazelnut flour
- ½ cup flax flour
- ½ cup pumpkin seeds
- ½ cup sunflower seeds
- 2 eggs

Directions:

1. You can prepare the dough in the same way as described in the previous recipe.
2. Preheat the oven to 0°C (425°F).
3. In a bowl, beat the eggs by a mixer until dense mass, and add flour and seeds. Mix it all again.
4. Cover the baking sheet with parchment. Lay out the dough.
5. Bake in the oven for 10 minutes. Cut into the desired number of sticks and put on the switched-off oven for 20 minutes.

Nutrition Info: Per Servings: Calories: 88 Fats: 14 g Carbs: 2.1 g Proteins: 15 g

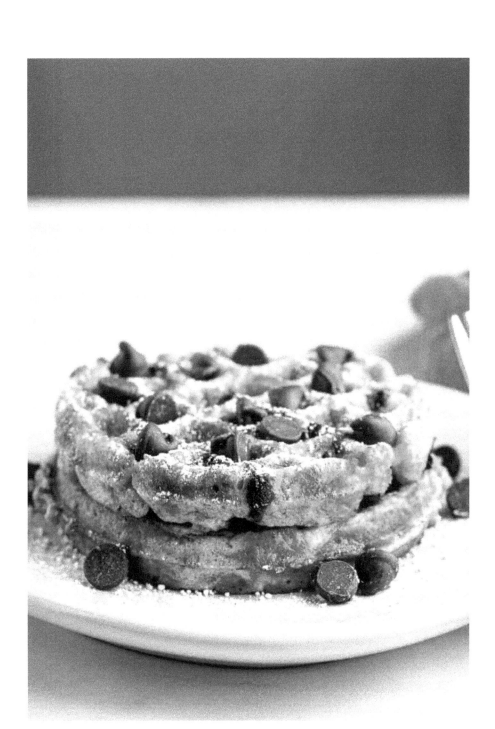

Keto Waffles

Servings: 3

Cooking Time: 30 Minutes

Ingredients:

- For the Ketogenic waffles:
- 8 Oz of cream cheese
- 5 Large pastured eggs
- 1/3 Cup of coconut flour
- ½ Teaspoon of Xanthan gum
- 1 Pinch of salt
- ½ Teaspoon of vanilla extract
- 2 Tablespoons of Swerve
- ¼ Teaspoon of baking soda
- 1/3 Cup of almond milk
- Optional ingredients:
- ½ Teaspoon of cinnamon pie spice
- ¼ Teaspoon of almond extract
- To prepare the low-carb Maple Syrup:
- 1 Cup of water
- 1 Tablespoon of Maple flavour
- ¾ Cup of powdered Swerve
- 1 Tablespoon of almond butter
- ½ Teaspoon of Xanthan gum

Directions:

1. For the waffles:
2. Make sure all your ingredients are exactly at room temperature.
3. Place all your ingredients for the waffles from cream cheese to pastured eggs, coconut flour, Xanthan gum, salt, vanilla extract, the Swerve, the baking soda and the almond milk except for the almond milk with the help of a processor.
4. Blend your ingredients until it becomes smooth and creamy; then transfer the batter to a bowl.
5. Add the almond milk and mix your ingredients with a spatula.
6. Heat a waffle maker to a temperature of high.
7. Spray your waffle maker with coconut oil and add about ¼ of the batter in it evenly with a spatula into your waffle iron.
8. Close your waffle and cook until you get the colour you want.
9. Carefully remove the waffles to a platter.
10. For the Ketogenic Maple Syrup:
11. Place 1 and ¼ cups of water, the swerve and the maple in a small pan and bring to a boil over a low heat; then let simmer for about 10 minutes.
12. Add the coconut oil.
13. Sprinkle the Xanthan gum over the top of the waffle and use an immersion blender to blend smoothly.

14. Serve and enjoy your delicious waffles!

Nutrition Info: Calories: 316;Fat: 26g;Carbohydrates: 7g;Fiber: 3g;Protein: 11g

Garlic Bread

Servings: 10

Cooking Time: 20 Minutes

Ingredients:

- 1 package bread baking mass
- 1 ⅓ cup warm water
- 1 tbsp butter
- 3 garlic cloves
- 1 tbsp dry oregano

Directions:

1. In a bowl, mix the dough from the bread baking mass and water. Make a long baguette.
2. Cover the baking sheet with parchment. Place the baguette on the baking sheet and make shallow notches.
3. Bake in the oven at a temperature of 180°C (6°F) for 25 minutes.
4. Prepare the garlic butter. Mix the butter, chopped garlic, and oregano.
5. Grate hot bread with garlic butter and send to the oven for 10 minutes.

Nutrition Info: Per Servings: Calories: 80 Fats: 15 g Carbs: 1.g Proteins: 9 g

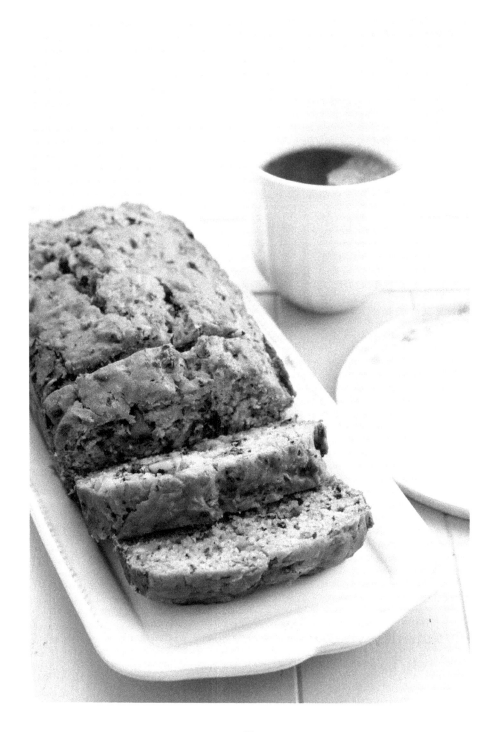

Bread With Zucchini And Walnuts

Servings: 12

Cooking Time: 85 Minutes

Ingredients:

- 1 cup almond flour
- 1 zucchini
- 3 eggs
- 1 tbsp erythritol
- 2 tbsp walnuts
- 3 tbsp olive oil
- 1 tsp vanilla
- 1 tsp baking powder
- 1 tsp cinnamon
- ½ tsp ginger powder
- A pinch of salt

Directions:

1. The oven to be preheated to 0°C (356°F).
2. In a bowl, mix the eggs, butter, and vanilla. In another container, mix the flour, sweetener, baking powder, cinnamon, ginger powder, and salt.
3. Chop the zucchini until uniformity. Drain excess liquid.
4. Add the dry ingredients and zucchini to the egg. Beat them by a mixer for 1 minute until uniformity.

5. Lay out the dough into the greased form. Decorate with chopped walnuts.

Nutrition Info: Per Servings: Calories: 123 Fats: 15.3 g Carbs: 4.8 g Proteins: 6 g

Flax Seed Crackers

Servings: 25

Cooking Time: 10 Minutes

Ingredients:

- 2 and 1/2 cups of almond flour
- ½ Cup of coconut flour
- 1 Teaspoon of ground flaxseed meal
- ½ Teaspoon of dried rosemary, chopped
- ½ Teaspoon of onion powder
- ¼ Teaspoon of kosher salt
- 3 large organic eggs
- 1 Tablespoon of extra-virgin olive oil

Directions:

1. Preheat your oven to a temperature of about 325 F.
2. Line a baking sheet with a parchment paper.
3. In a large bowl; combine the flours with the rosemary, the flax meal, the salt and the onion powder and mix.
4. Crack in the eggs and add the oil; then mix very well and combine your ingredients very well.
5. Keep mixing until you get the shape of a large ball for about 1 minute.
6. Cut the dough into the 2 pieces of parchment paper and roll it to a thickness of about ¼".

7. Cut the dough into squares and transfer it to the prepared baking sheet.

8. Bake your dough for about 13 to 15 minutes; then let cool for about 15 minutes.

9. Serve and enjoy your crackers or store in a container.

Nutrition Info: Calories: 150.2;Fat: 13g;Carbohydrates: 5.4g;Fiber: 2.6g;Protein: 7g

Keto Blender Buns

Servings:6

Cooking Time: 25 Minutes

Ingredients:

- 4 Whole Eggs
- ¼ cup Melted Butter
- ½ tsp Salt
- ½ cup Almond Flour
- 1 tsp Italian Spice Mix

Directions:

1. Preheat oven to 425F.
2. Pulse all ingredients in a blender.
3. Divide batter into a 6-hole muffin tin.
4. Bake for 25 minutesutes.

Nutrition Info: Per Servings: Fat: 18 g. Protein: 8 g. Carbs: 2 g.

Buffalo Chicken Sausage Balls

Servings: 12

Cooking Time: 25 Minutes

Ingredients:

- Sausage Balls:
- 2 14-ox sausages, casings removed
- 2 cups almond flour
- 1 ½ cups shredded cheddar cheese
- ½ cup crumbled bleu cheese
- 1 tsp salt
- ½ tsp pepper
- Bleu Cheese Ranch Dipping Sauce:
- 1/3 cup mayonnaise
- 1/3 cup almond milk, unsweetened
- 2 cloves garlic, minced
- 1 tsp dried dill
- ½ tsp dried parsley
- ½ tsp salt
- ½ tsp pepper
- ¼ cup crumbled bleu cheese (or more, if desired)

Directions:

1. Preheat your oven at 350 degrees F.
2. Layer two baking sheets with wax paper and set them aside.

3. Mix sausage with cheddar cheese, almond flour, salt, pepper, and bleu cheese in a large bowl.
4. Make 1-inch balls out of this mixture and place them on the baking sheets.
5. Bake them for 2minutes until golden brown.
6. Meanwhile, prepare the dipping sauce by whisking all of its ingredients in a bowl.
7. Serve the balls with this dipping sauce.

Nutrition Info: Calories 1 Total Fat 15 g Saturated Fat 12.1 g Cholesterol 11 mg Sodium 31 mg Total Carbs 6.2 g Sugar 1.6 g Fiber 0.8 g Protein 4.5 g

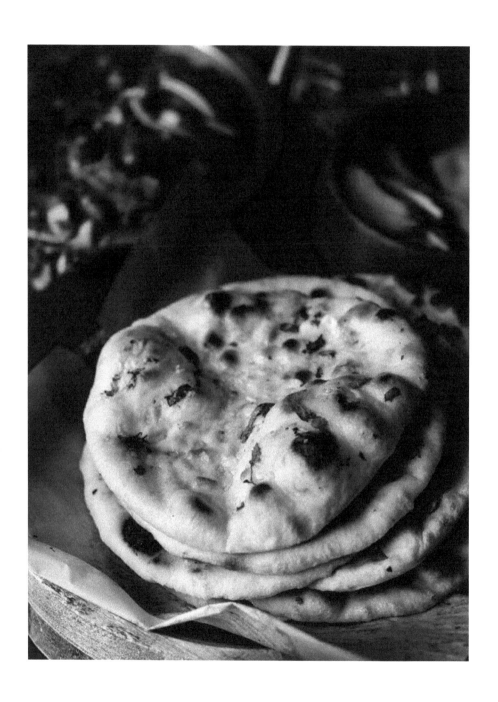

Indian Bread With Greens

Servings: 6-8

Cooking Time: 75 Minutes

Ingredients:

- ⅔ cup coconut flour
- 2 tbsp psyllium
- ½ cup coconut oil
- 2 ½ tbsp bran
- 1 ½ tsp baking powder
- 2 cups water
- ½ tsp salt
- A bunch of fresh cilantro
- ¼ cup butter

Directions:

1. Mix all dry ingredients, and add melted coconut oilin abowl. Boil water, add to the mass and knead the dough. Leave it for 5 minutes.
2. Divide the dough into 8 round pieces. Roll out each piece into a thin flat cake. Fry in a pan with coconut oil.
3. Put flat cakes on a plate. Melt the butter, and chop the cilantro. Lubricate bread by butter and sprinkle with greens.

Nutrition Info: Per Servings: Calories: 9 Fats: 17 g Carbs: 4.6 g Proteins: 4.5 g

Buns With Yogurt And Seeds

Servings: 6

Cooking Time: 40 Minutes

Ingredients:

- ⅔ cup yogurt
- 1 cup almond flour
- 2 tbsp coconut flour
- 2 tbsp psyllium
- 4 eggs
- 3 tbsp + 1 tsp flax seeds (for decoration)
- 3 tbsp sunflower seeds
- 1 tsp baking powder
- ½ tsp salt

Directions:

1. The oven to be preheated to 5°C (365°F).
2. In a bowl, beat the eggs by a mixer until dense mass. Add yogurt, dry ingredients. Mix again. Leave the dough for 10 minutes.
3. Cover the baking sheet with parchment. Make the round buns and lay out them on a baking sheet.
4. Sprinkle with sunflower seeds and bake in the oven for 25 minutes.

Nutrition Info: Per Servings: Calories: 10 Fats: 15 g Carbs: 3.6 g Proteins: 16 g

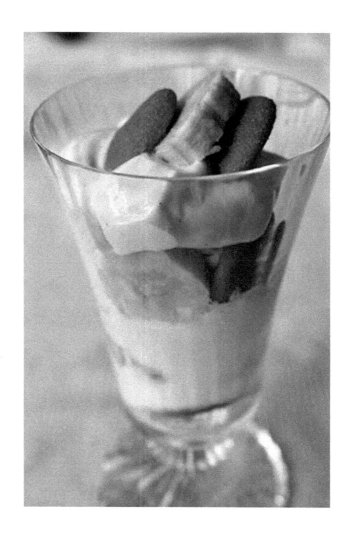

Citrus Bread

Servings: 10

Cooking Time: 20 Minutes

Ingredients:

- ½ cup almond flour
- 3 tbsp dried cherry
- 1 egg
- 3 tbsp almonds
- 2 tbsp coconut oil
- 1 tbsp liquid stevia
- ⅓ tsp baking powder
- 1 tsp grapefruit peel
- ¼ cup grapefruit juice
- Salt to taste

Directions:

1. The oven to be preheated to 0°C (356°F).
2. In a bowl, mix coconut oil, egg and grapefruit juice. Chop the cherries and almonds.
3. In another bowl, mix the flour, sweetener, baking powder, almonds, cherry, grapefruit peel, and salt. Add the egg mass. Mix well.
4. Lay out the prepared dough in a greased cake form. For 25 minutes bake until crust.

Nutrition Info: Per Servings: Calories: 7 Fats: 7.9 g Carbs: 3.9 g Proteins: 7.3 g

Buns With Cheese And Sesame

Servings: 8

Cooking Time: 50 Minutes

Ingredients:

- 3 eggs
- 2 tbsp coconut flour
- 2 tbsp almond flour
- ¼ cup butter
- ⅔ cup sour cream
- ¾ cup + 1 tbsp grated parmesan
- 2 tbsp psyllium
- 2 tsp baking powder
- 1 tsp sesame seeds
- ½ tsp salt

Directions:

1. The oven to be preheated to 0°C (375°F).
2. Melt the butter on a water bath or in a microwave. In a bowl, beat the eggs by a mixer for minutes until uniformity. Add butter and sour cream. Mix again.
3. Add grated parmesan and dry ingredients, mix until uniformity. Leave the dough for 10 minutes.
4. Make the buns and lay out them on a baking sheet covered with a parchment. Sprinkle with parmesan. Bake in the oven for 25 minutes.

Nutrition Info: Per Servings: Calories: 1 Fats: 27 g Carbs: 1.9 g Proteins: 15 g

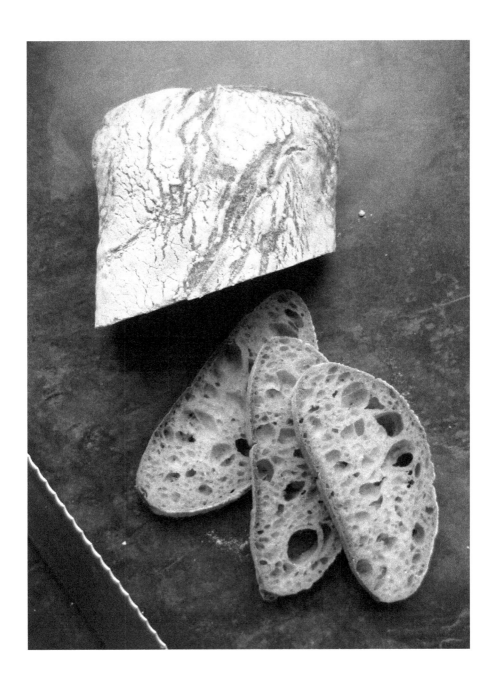

Keto Ciabatta

Servings:8

Cooking Time: 30 Minutes

Ingredients:

- 1 cup Almond Flour
- ¼ cup Psyllium Husk Powder
- ½ tsp Salt
- 1 tsp Baking Powder
- 3 tbsp Olive Oil
- 1 tsp Maple Syrup
- 1 tbsp Active Dry Yeast
- 1 cup Warm Water
- 1 tbsp Chopped Rosemary

Directions:

1. In a bowl, stir together warm water, maple syrup, and yeast. Leave for minutes.
2. In a separate bowl, whisk together almond flour, psyllium husk powder, salt, chopped rosemary, and baking powder.
3. Stir in the olive oil and yeast mixture into the dry ingredients until a smooth dough is formed.
4. Knead the dough until smooth.
5. Divide the dough.

6. Set both buns on a baking sheet lined with parchment. Leave to rise for an hour.

7. Bake for 30 minutes at 380F.

Nutrition Info: Per Servings: Fat: 11 g. Protein: 3 g. Carbs: 4 g.

Peanut Butter Granola

Servings: 12

Cooking Time: 30 Minutes

Ingredients:

- 1 ½ cups almonds
- 1 ½ cups pecans
- 1 cup shredded coconut
- ¼ cup sunflower seeds
- 1/3 cup Swerve sweetener
- 1/3 cup vanilla whey protein powder
- 1/3 cup peanut butter
- ¼ cup butter
- ¼ cup water

Directions:

1. Preheat your oven at 300 degrees F.
2. Layer a baking sheet with wax paper and set it aside.
3. Add almonds and pecans to a food processor and finely grind them.
4. Add coconut, protein powder, sweetener, and sunflower seeds to the nut mixture in a bowl.
5. Add butter and peanut butter to another bowl and melt it in the microwave by heating for 30 sec or 1 minute.
6. Mix well then pour it into the nut mixture.

7. After mixing it up, spread this mixture on a baking sheet in an even layer.

8. Bake for 30 minutes then allow it to cool.

9. Serve.

Nutrition Info: Calories Total Fat 15.5 g Saturated Fat 4.5 g Cholesterol 12 mg Sodium 18 mg Total Carbs 4.4 g Sugar 1.2 g Fiber 0.3 g Protein 4.8 g

Juicy Blueberry Muffins

Servings: 6

Cooking Time: 20 Minutes

Ingredients:

- 1 cup Almond Flour
- 1 pinch Salt
- ⅛ tsp Baking Soda
- 1 Egg
- 2 Tbsp Coconut Oil, melted
- ½ cup Coconut Milk
- ¼ cup Fresh Blueberries

Directions:

1. Preheat your oven to 350F 5C.
2. Set aside after combining.
3. In another bowl, whisk the egg, coconut oil, coconut milk. And add the mix to the almond flour mixture. Mix gently to incorporate but do not overmix.
4. Gently mix in the blueberries and fill the cupcakes with the batter.
5. Once baked and golden brown, remove from the oven, allow to cool before serving after baking for 20-2minutes.

Nutrition Info: Per Servings: Calories: 1.8, Total Fat: 15.1 g, Saturated Fat: 5.3 g, Carbs: 5.5 g, Sugars: 1.8 g, Protein: 5.2 g

Bread With Cottage Cheese

Servings: 10

Cooking Time: 65 Minutes

Ingredients:

- 1 ¼ cup almond flour
- ⅔ cup natural yogurt
- 5 oz cottage cheese
- 6 eggs
- 2 tbsp flax seeds
- 2 tbsp sesame seeds
- 2 tbsp psyllium
- 2 tsp baking powder
- A pinch of salt

Directions:

1. The oven to be preheated to 0°C (356°F).
2. In another bowl, beat the eggs; add yogurt, and cottage cheese. Mix contents of two bowls. Leave the dough for 10 minutes.
3. Grease the bread baking form and lay out the dough into it. Level out with a spoon.
4. Bake in a hot oven for 50 minutes.

Nutrition Info: Per Servings: Calories: 6 Fats: 6.1 g Carbs: 2.6 g Proteins: 11 g

Nuts Buns With Cheese

Servings: 6-8

Cooking Time: 35 Minutes

Ingredients:

- ½ cup almond flour
- ¼ cup sesame seeds
- ¼ cup sunflower seeds
- 1 tbsp psyllium
- 3 eggs
- 1 ½ cup grated cheese
- 1 tsp baking powder

Directions:

1. The oven to be preheated to 200°C (400°F).
2. In a bowl, beat the eggs by a mixer until dense mass. Add cheese and dry ingredients, mix well. Leave the dough for 10 minutes.
3. Cover the baking sheet with parchment. Make the small buns and lay out them on a baking sheet.
4. Bake in the oven for 18 minutes.

Nutrition Info: Per Servings: Calories: 102 Fats: 14.1 g Carbs: 2.6 g Proteins: 20 g

Buns With Cream Cheese And Cinnamon

Servings: 12

Cooking Time: 40 Minutesutes

Ingredients:

- for the dough:
- ¾ cup almond flour
- 1 egg
- 2 tbsp cream cheese
- ½ tsp baking powder
- 5.5 oz of mozzarella
- for filling:
- 2 tbsp cream cheese
- 3 tbsp stevia
- 2 tbsp water
- 2 tsp cinnamon

Directions:

1. The oven to be preheated to 0°C (356°F).
2. Grind the mozzarella. Add the cream cheese and heat in the microwave for minutesutes. Add the flour, baking powder and egg to the cheese mass.
3. Mix well and knead the elastic dough. Divide into 8 round balls. Pull each part out into a long sausage and roll it out.

4. Prepare the filling. In a bowl, mix 2 tablespoons stevia, cinnamon and water. Pour the filling on the dough. Form the tight sausage and cut into 10-12 buns.

5. Put the buns on a baking sheet with parchment and bake in the oven for 2minutesutes.

6. Mix the cream cheese and 1 tbsp stevia. Lubricate hot buns with creamy dressing.

Nutrition Info: Per Servings: Calories: 81 Fats: 11 g Carbs: 3.5 g Proteins: 10 g

Garlic Buns

Servings: 10

Cooking Time: 65 Minutes

Ingredients:

- ½ cup almond flour
- 3 egg whites
- 5 tbsp psyllium
- ½ cup butter
- 2 tsp baking powder
- ½ tsp salt
- 1 tbsp sesame seeds
- ⅓ cup of boiled water
- 2 garlic cloves
- 2 tsp balsamic vinegar

Directions:

1. Preheat the ovent to 0°C (356°F).
2. Add whipped egg whites, vinegar, chopped garlic, and boiled water. Mix mass by a mixer for 1 minutesute.
3. Make the round buns with wet hands and lay out them on the baking sheet. Grease buns with melted butter and sprinkle with sesame seeds. Ensure that it is baked for minutes.

Nutrition Info: Per Servings: Calories: 95 Fats: 9 g Carbs: 3 g Proteins: 2 g

Blueberry Scones

Servings: 12

Cooking Time: 25 Minutes

Ingredients:

- 2 cups almond flour
- 1/3 cup Swerve sweetener
- ¼ cup coconut flour
- 1 tbsp baking powder
- ¼ tsp salt
- 2 large eggs
- ¼ cup heavy whipping cream
- ½ tsp vanilla extract
- ¾ cup fresh blueberries

Directions:

1. Preheat your oven at 325 degrees F. Layer a baking sheet with wax paper.
2. Whisk almond flour with baking powder, salt, coconut flour, and sweetener in a large bowl.
3. Stir in eggs, vanilla, and cream then mix well until fully incorporated.
4. Add blueberries and mix gently.
5. Spread this dough on a baking sheet and form it into a 10x8-inch rectangle.

6. Slice the dough into equal-sized squares then cut each diagonally to make triangles.

7. Arrange these triangles on the baking sheet 1 inch apart from each other.

8. Bake these scones for 25 minutes until golden.

9. Allow them to cool then serve.

Nutrition Info: Calories 266 Total Fat 25.7 g Saturated Fat 1.2 g Cholesterol 41 mg Sodium 18 mg Total Carbs 9.7 g Sugar 1.2 g Fiber 0.5 g Protein 2.6 g

Sticks Grissini With Chia And Cheese

Servings: 15

Cooking Time: 40 Minutes

Ingredients:

- 5 tbsp chia seeds
- 1 tbsp psyllium
- 2 oz cheddar
- 2 tbsp cold water
- 1 tbsp olive oil
- 1 tbsp dried oregano
- A pinch of salt

Directions:

1. The oven to be preheated to 0°C (375°F).
2. Grate the cheddar on a small grater. In a deep bowl, mix psyllium, chia seeds, cheese, oregano, and salt. Add olive oil and water. Knead the dense dough.
3. Cover the baking sheet with parchment. Roll the dough.
4. Cut into thin strips and put on the switched-off oven for another 5 minutes. Cool it down.

Nutrition Info: Per Servings: Calories: 93 Fats: 20 g Carbs: 2.1 g Proteins: 20.1 g

Homemade Graham Crackers

Servings: 12

Cooking Time: 30 Minutes

Ingredients:

- 2 cups almond flour
- 1/3 cup Swerve Brown
- 2 tsp cinnamon
- 1 tsp baking powder
- Pinch salt
- 1 large egg
- 2 tbsp butter, melted
- 1 tsp vanilla extract

Directions:

1. Preheat your oven at 300 degrees F.
2. Whisk almond flour, baking powder, salt, cinnamon, and sweetener in a large bowl.
3. Stir in melted butter, egg, and vanilla extract.
4. Mix well to form the dough then spread it out into a ¼-inch thick sheet.
5. Slice the sheet into 2x2-inch squares and place them on a baking sheet with wax paper.
6. Bake them for 30 minutes until golden then let them sit for 30 minutes at room temperature until cooled.

7. Break the crackers into smaller squares and put them back in the hot oven for 30 minutes. Keep the oven off during this time.

8. Enjoy.

Nutrition Info: Calories 243 Total Fat 21 g Saturated Fat 18.2 g Cholesterol 121 mg Sodium 34 mg Total Carbs 7.3 g Sugar 0.g Fiber 0.1 g Protein 4.3 g

Pumpkin Custard

Servings: 6

Cooking Time: 40 Minutes

Ingredients:

- 4 egg yolks
- ¾ cup coconut cream
- 18 tsp cloves
- 18 tsp ginger
- ½ tsp cinnamon
- 1 tsp liquid stevia
- 15 oz pumpkin puree

Directions:

1. Preheat the oven to 350 F 0 C.
2. In a large bowl, mix together pumpkin puree, cloves, ginger, cinnamon, and swerve.
3. Add egg yolks and beat until well combined.
4. Add coconut cream and stir well.
5. Pour mixture into the six ramekins.
6. Bake in preheated oven for 35-40 minutes.
7. Allow to cool completely then place in the refrigerator.
8. Serve chilled and enjoy.

Nutrition Info: Per Servings: Net Carbs: 5.2g; Calories: 130; Total Fat: 10.4g; Saturated Fat: 7.5g Protein: 3.3g; Carbs: 8g; Fiber: 2.8g; Sugar: 3.4g; Fat 73% Protein 11% Carbs 16%

Creamy Avocado Dessert

Servings: 4

Cooking Time: 0 Minutes

Ingredients:

- 1 avocado, peeled, pitted, and diced
- 1/4 cup heavy whipping cream
- Liquid stevia, to taste
- 1/4 teaspoon vanilla essence
- 1/4 teaspoon cinnamon, ground

Directions:

1. Beat everything in a food processor until smooth.
2. Transfer the yogurt mixture to a sealable bowl.
3. Place the mixture in the freezer for about 1 hour.
4. Serve and enjoy.

Nutrition Info: Calories 266 ;Total Fat 27 g ;Saturated Fat 1.2 g ;Cholesterol 41 mg ;Sodium 18 mg ;Total Carbs 9.7 g ;Sugar 1.2 g ;Fiber 0.5 g ;Protein 2.6 g

Chocolate Peanut Butter Popsicles

Servings: 4

Cooking Time: 0 Minute

Ingredients:

- 1/2 cup peanut butter
- 1 tsp liquid stevia
- 1.5 cups almond milk
- 1 cup heavy whipping cream
- 1/4 cup cocoa powder sugar free

Directions:

1. Beat all the ingredients together in a food processor until smooth.
2. Divide this mixture into the popsicle molds and insert the ice cream sticks in it.
3. Freeze them for about 4 hours or more.
4. Serve after removing from the molds.
5. Enjoy.

Nutrition Info: Per Servings: Calories 147 Total Fat 11 g Saturated Fat 10.1 g Cholesterol 10 mg Total Carbs 4.2 g Sugar 2 g Fiber 0.4 g Sodium 91 mg Potassium 48 mg Protein 3.2 g

Lemon Ice Cream

Servings: 6

Cooking Time: 5 Minutes

Ingredients:

- 1 lemon, juiced and zested
- 1/3 cup erythritol sweetener
- 3 eggs
- 1 ¾ cups heavy whipping cream, full-fat and unsweetened

Directions:

1. Separate egg yolks and white in two bowls and beat egg whites with an electric beater until stiff peaks form.
2. Add sweetener to egg yolks and whisk until light and fluffy.
3. Then stir in lemon juice and fold egg yolks into egg white.
4. Place cream in another bowl and whip well until soft peaks form.
5. Place the bowl in the freezer and freeze for 2 hours or until ice cream reach to the desired consistency, stirring every half an hour.
6. When ready to serve, thaw ice cream for 15 minutes at room temperature and then scoop into serving bowls.

Nutrition Info: Calories: 269 Cal, Carbs: 3 g, Fat: 2g, Protein: 5 g, Fiber: 0 g.

Strawberry Yogurt

Servings: 8

Cooking Time: 5 Minutes

Ingredients:

- 4 cups frozen strawberries
- 12 cup plain yogurt
- 1 tsp liquid stevia
- 1 tbsp fresh lemon juice

Directions:

1. Add all ingredients into the blender and blend until yogurt is smooth and creamy.
2. Serve immediately and enjoy.

Nutrition Info: Per Servings: Net Carbs: 6.1g; Calories: ; Total Fat: 0.9g; Saturated Fat: 0.2g Protein: 1g; Carbs: 7.6g; Fiber: 1.5g; Sugar: 5.6g; Fat 22% Protein 11% Carbs 67%

Cocoa Yogurt Ice Cream

Servings: 4

Cooking Time: 0 Minutes

Ingredients:

- 2½ oz. fat-free Greek yogurt
- ½ oz. vanilla protein powder
- 1 teaspoon unsweetened cocoa powder
- ½ cup unsweetened almond milk
- 1 teaspoon vanilla essence
- Stevia to taste
- Almonds & berries (optional)

Directions:

1. Beat everything in a food processor until smooth.
2. Transfer the yogurt mixture to a sealable bowl.
3. Place the mixture in the freezer for about 4 hours.
4. During this time, churn this ice cream in an ice cream maker after every 30 minutes.
5. Garnish with berries and almonds.
6. Serve.

Nutrition Info: Calories 11;Total Fat 21.2 g ;Saturated Fat 10.4 g ;Cholesterol 19.7 mg ;Sodium 104 mg ;Total Carbs 7.3 g ;Sugar 3.4 g ;Fiber 2 g ;Protein 8.1 g

Fudge Popsicles

Servings: 4

Cooking Time: 0 Minute

Ingredients:

- 1 3/4 cup heavy cream
- 2 1/2 ounces sugar free chocolate, chopped
- 1/3 cup erythritol blend
- 2 large eggs
- 3/4 cup almond milk
- 1 teaspoon vanilla essence

Directions:

1. Mix heavy cream with chocolate, eggs, and sweetener in a saucepan.
2. Let this mixture simmer on low heat then remove it instantly.
3. Stir in vanilla essence and almond milk. Mix well.
4. Pour this mixture into suitable popsicle molds and insert ice cream sticks in it.
5. Freeze them for hours or more.
6. Remove the popsicles from the molds.
7. Serve.

Nutrition Info: Per Servings: Calories 117 Total Fat 21.2 g Saturated Fat 10.4 g Cholesterol 19.7 mg Total Carbs 7.3 g

Sugar 3.4 g Fiber 2 g Sodium 104 mg Potassium 196 mg Protein 1 g

Saffron Pannacotta

Servings: 6

Cooking Time: 2 Hours And 10 Minutes

Ingredients:

- ½ tablespoon gelatin
- 1 tablespoon swerve sweetener
- ¼ teaspoon vanilla extract, unsweetened
- 1/16 teaspoon saffron
- 2 cups heavy whipping cream, full-fat
- Water as needed
- 1 tablespoon chopped almonds, toasted

Directions:

1. Place gelatin in a small bowl and stir in small amount of water according to instructions on the pack, or tablespoon water for 1 teaspoon of gelatin and set aside until bloom.
2. In the meantime, place a small saucepan over medium heat, add remaining ingredients except for almonds, stir well and bring the mixture to a light boil.
3. Then lower heat and simmer mixture for minutes or until mixture begin to thicken.
4. Remove pan from heat, stir in gelatin until dissolved completely and divide the mixture evenly between six ramekins.

5. Cover ramekins with plastic wrap and chill in the refrigerator for 2 hours.

6. When ready to serve, top with toasted almonds and serve.

Nutrition Info: Calories: 2 Cal, Carbs: 2 g, Fat: 29 g, Protein: 3 g, Fiber: 0 g.

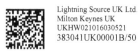

Lightning Source UK Ltd.
Milton Keynes UK
UKHW021016030521
383041UK00001B/50